Pregnancy

Holistic Women' s Guide Book to A Healthy Pregnancy

Table of Contents

Introduction

I want to thank you and congratulate you for downloading the book, *"Pregnancy: Holistic Women's Guide Book to a Healthy Pregnancy."*

This book contains proven steps and strategies on how to go through your pregnancy in a **healthy and natural way**, avoiding exposure to potentially negative influences that can harm you or the baby throughout your pregnancy. By using natural treatments, healthy habits, and nutritional guidance, you can have the best pregnancy possible for both you and your baby!

Many times during pregnancy, women feel that the doctor is not on their side. The doctor may ignore some of their symptoms, or try to placate them with prescription medicines that aren't that good for them, and may not really deal with the issues they are having in the pregnancy.

A holistic approach is **much better**. While it doesn't necessarily avoid medication, it carefully looks at all the angles of the problem to find the solution that is right for you and for the baby. For example, you may come in with complaints of a backache. Your regular doctor may prescribe aspirin or another painkiller that can be toxic for you and the baby. A holistic approach doctor would first recommend hot compresses, massage, and some light exercise with stretching to help the back feel better.

This and many other issues are discussed in this guide, and you will see that it is geared towards a pregnancy experience resulting in **confident, healthy and happy mothers**, awaiting the arrival of healthier and happier babies.

Holistic health is not something to be scared or fearful of. It is a **natural way** to take care of your body and your baby without feeling like the decisions made are potentially more about feeding the economic pipeline of the traditional medical and pharmaceutical industries.

If you are interested in finding out more about holistic pregnancy concepts, make sure to read through this book in its entirety. We go into detail on many aspects of holistic pregnancy care, such as **herbal supplementation**, which will provide extra support for your body and will keep you healthy through all parts of your pregnancy.

The holistic approach keeps **YOU** in mind and helps you to achieve the very best pregnancy possible. Take some time to read through this guide to learn as much as possible about this natural and ultimately rewarding approach to pregnancy and childbirth.

Thanks again for downloading this book, I hope will you enjoy it!

information is without contract or any type of guarantee assurance.

The trademarks that are used are without any consent, and the publication of the trademark is without permission or backing by the trademark owner. All trademarks and brands within this book are for clarifying purposes only and are the owned by the owners themselves, not affiliated with this document.

Chapter 1:
Understanding Holistic Medicine
& the Holistic Approach

To get started, we should take a look at holistic medicine. This type of medicine often gets a bad name. People feel that it may not work as well as pharmaceutical medicine, and that it can't do a good job in helping you to stay healthy or have a good pregnancy experience. The abundance of misinformation about holistic medicine is undoubtedly a contributing factor to the negative stereotypes.

Holistic medicine is the science and art of healing that does not just focus on the problem at hand, but addresses the whole person. The holistic approach considers the physical, social, spiritual and psychological aspects. This practice combines alternative and conventional therapies in the hope of treating and preventing disease and promoting the optimal health of the patient.

Many people have been misled about holistic medicine. The pharmaceutical industry has worked hard to take over the market, convincing many new mothers that the holistic realm is bad for them and their baby. The holistic approach is not something that is radical and there may be times you will still need to use prescribed medicine to help out with your condition. Rather than feeding your body chemicals that may not be needed, the holistic approach takes things a step further and finds the right treatment, whether it is a healthy diet, a change in physical activity, counseling.

The advantage to this approach is the inherent objectivity it brings. A holistic doctor will not pick a treatment because it is the easiest or because he is going to make a lot of money from the medication that is prescribed. Instead, he will design the healthiest option for you in order to allow the life force to flow through your body unimpeded, so your spirit, mind, and body feel as good as possible.

While traditional doctors in clinical settings are pressured to quickly prescribe a solution to address the symptoms of each patient and move to the next on a very tight schedule, the holistic approach is focused on fixing the underlying problem. The holistic approach looks at your past history to determine what needs to happen to make your body start working correctly again. Masking the symptoms doesn't help in the long run and could make the situation worse.

For holistic medicine to work, you need to be an active participant in the treatment. You have to work with the doctor to determine the best treatment for your needs. Answering their questions, being honest, and working towards a solution that is good for the whole body, mind, and spirit can help you to improve not only your physical symptoms, but other area of your life as well. This process may be more time consuming and hard to go through, but it really is the best way to ensure that you are getting the right treatment to actually take care of your condition without side effects or causing another problem.

Finding a doctor who uses this kind of approach is not always the easiest thing to achieve. Many doctors are under strict time constraints, trying to take care of too many patients in a short amount of time. Ask around to make sure that you find the right holistic medicine practitioner that will actually commit the time to listen to you and find a treatment that works for the whole body, rather than turning first to a medication that may just hide the problem.

Principles of Holistic Medicine

The first thing that we need to look at in order to determine what holistic medicine is all about and how it can help out every aspect of your health, beyond just the disease or condition that is affecting you at the moment, is to look at some of the principles that go along with holistic medicine. Holistic medicine is a practice that believes that unconditional support and love is one of the best natural healers available, and that the patient plays a critical role in providing reliable information to the doctor and then faithfully implementing the treatment plan identified.

Some of the other principles that come with the holistic approach include:

- Every person has healing powers inside of them that they can use to their advantage.

- The patient is not defined by their disease and should not be treated this way.

- To find the right healing for each person, it takes a team. The patient and the doctor will need to work together to address all parts of the patients life to determine the right course of action to make things better.

- Treatment must involve finding how to fix the root cause of a condition or disease, rather than just getting rid of the symptoms.

When all of these things come into play, you are going to get some of the best care in the world. Many patients may not realize how great this process is for their whole body. They may be taking medicine from their doctors and assuming that since the pain or discomfort has gone away that the problem is fixed. Unfortunately, most medications and treatments are just temporary and are numbing you to the real underlying issue. As soon as the medication wears off, you will go back to experiencing the same issue again.

With the holistic approach, the condition's root is addressed and the patient is not seen as just another number. You will find a good treatment, one that actually works on the body and is best for you. This is so important when you are pregnant. To find a treatment that works the best for you and for the baby, and considers the reality that every pregnancy is unique, is the best way to ensure that the pregnancy will go as smoothly as possible.

Chapter 2:
Preparing for Motherhood

Now that we know a little bit more about holistic medicine, it is time to work on preparing yourself for motherhood. This is an exciting time in your life and can begin even before you conceive. You could be working on getting pregnant and preparing your body, and your life, for the joy of becoming a mother. It is a big decision, but one that you will cherish forever. Providing a safe environment for the baby will help the pregnancy go well and the baby to be as healthy as can be.

There has been recent research that discovered that the nutrients found in the environment of your growing fetus will play a huge role in their genetic expression. The baby's risk of disease and their overall health are at least partly dependent on the nutrient intake and the health of the mother not only during the pregnancy, but also before and after the birth of the baby.

Both the father and the mother should work on improving their health before they even try to conceive. When the mother gets pregnant, the baby will have access to the nutrients in her body, even before she discovers she is pregnant. If the mother is low on a particular nutrient, the baby will be taking in all the reserves in the mother's body for that nutrient. The baby will not suffer unless there is a huge deficiency in the nutrient; but the mother will be deficient which will take a toll on her, and eventually impact the baby if the issue is not addressed in time.

In order to ensure that the mother and the baby have enough nutrients during the pregnancy, the mother needs to get on a good nutritional plan so she gets plenty of great vitamins and nutrients that are needed to stay healthy. The father should go on this kind of diet as well. While he won't be carrying the baby during pregnancy, having good health will promote him to be in an optimal mental and physical state for taking care of the child and the mother.

It is recommended that both parents start eating a proper nutritious diet 6 to 12 months before you plan on conceiving if possible. You should take in plenty of zinc and folic acid as well, since these vitamins and minerals are going to help with detoxing the body and increase fertility.

Of course, conceiving is not always something that is planned, at least not 12 months in advance. Many doctors do recommend that women who are in their reproductive prime years eat a healthy diet and consider taking a prenatal vitamin just to be on the safe side. This way, if they do become pregnant without the time to get prepared, they are still going to have enough of the important necessary nutrients to keep the baby healthy.

Steps to Prepare for Pregnancy

1. Make your mental health a priority

   Share any history of mental health problems with your care provider. Recognize the extra stressors and hormonal influence that are a normal part of pregnancy and incorporate that into your treatment plan.

2. Clean up your diet

   This is a great time to implement a healthy diet and regular exercise program. Eliminate processed foods, and incorporate healthy and natural whole foods such as fruits and vegetables. Try to eat organically grown and local if possible.

3. Limit the toxins

   Reduce contact with the toxins found in chemicals you are exposed to, and be aware of toxic environments. Educate yourself on this topic so you can limit exposure to unnatural chemicals found in mainstream soaps, cleaners, cosmetics, etc.

4. Reduce the stress

   Stress can be very hard on your body and it can make it more difficult to get pregnant because cortisol levels that are high will suppress your ovulation, decrease the sex drive, and lower the sperm count.

   While some amount of stress is inevitable, learning to deal with it in a healthy way is the best thing you can do for your baby. Some suggestions for dealing with high levels of tension and stress are:

   - Taking a bath to calm down and relax.

   - Reading and escaping into a good story will take your mind off of your stress trigger.

   - Journaling and writing.

   - Exercise – even a little walking can make a big difference during pregnancy.

   - A support group, be it a formal group or simply friends and family. Choose a positive support system, and distance yourself from negative or toxic personalities.

- Get enough sleep – even a ten minute daytime nap can make a difference, and good sleeping habits will help you get restorative sleep. Set and keep a regular bedtime.

- Spend some time in nature, mother earth has all our answers.

- Get a professional body massage.

- Visualization.

- Breathing exercises.

- Meditation.

- Yoga – only go with poses that are approved for pregnancy.

If you have another method of relaxation that works for you, such as listening to some music, watching a funny show, or hanging out with loved ones, go ahead and do that as well. The activity is not as important as getting rid of the stress, as long as you do so in a healthy and safe way for you and your baby, before and during your pregnancy.

5. Acupuncture

Acupuncture is another great way to get your body ready for a new pregnancy. It can do so many great things for the whole body, but you do need to make sure that you are using someone who is certified and won't cause any damage to the body or make it harder to conceive. Some of the ways that acupuncture can help your body include:

- Improves how well in-vitro fertilization works.

- Helps induce relaxed states of mind while reducing the amount of stress felt.

- Increases how much blood gets to the uterus and can increase how thick the lining of the uterus is.

- Regulates your hormones so they produce more follicles.

- Improves how well the ovaries function so you get a healthier egg.

While you may have never tried acupuncture in the past, giving it a try can provide all of these benefits and more, making it easier than ever to be healthy for your pregnancy.

6. Get rid of negative thoughts

    Your mind is a powerful tool, and if you aren't careful, those negative thoughts could become self-fulfilling prophecies. Do not worry about the failures that you have had in the past. Do not listen to the negative stories that people are telling you or what you hear in the media. Throw those negative thoughts out because they just make you nervous and erode the best environment for a healthy pregnancy.

    Replace these thoughts with something positive. Think about how great it is going to be when you become pregnant. Think about anything that makes you happy or reminds you of something positive, and push those negative thoughts as far away as possible.

7. Trust in divine timing

It can be really frustrating to want to become pregnant and to find month after month that you are not expecting. But if you start to feel down about this, you are letting the negative thoughts come in. Rather, believe in divine timing. Things are going to happen when they are meant to happen. Maybe you just aren't ready for the child. Perhaps life has another plan for you and your child and you need to wait just a little longer. Plus, if you release some of this stress and let things naturally flow, rather than getting upset that it isn't working and having expectations, you are going to be pleasantly surprised once it finally happens.

8. See your dentist

While this may not be the first thing on your list, it is still important to make a visit to the dentist before you get pregnant and to keep your appointments even during pregnancy. During the pregnancy, the gums are more likely to bleed and your teeth can even become loose. If you are suffering from periodontal disease, you could have a higher risk of underweight or preterm babies, so keeping up with your dental appointments is critical, as all points of your pregnancy.

There are a few things that you can do in addition to visiting the dentist that will help to keep the teeth and gums healthy. First, take in lots of vitamin C as this is shown to provide healthier gums during pregnancy.

You should eat foods that are high in vitamin C, such as broccoli, red peppers, cabbage, tomatoes, strawberries, cantaloupe, kiwi, grapefruits, and oranges. Eat these foods fresh rather than canned to ensure that you are getting the full amount of nutrients without extra sugar and preservatives.

Vitamin A, vitamin E and folic acid are good as well. These nutrients are shown to reduce how much periodontal inflammation will occur during pregnancy, so work on getting lots of these into the diet. To get enough vitamin A into the diet, ingest plenty of kale, spinach, pumpkin, sweet potatoes, carrots, apricots, and mangos in your diet. Vitamin E can be found in almonds, spinach, sunflower seeds, chard, and mustard greens so eat up on these during pregnancy. To avoid gum disease, find better alternatives to sugary snacks, such as fruit.

9. Get some exercise

It is best to get started on an exercise routine before you get pregnant to prevent injuries. If you do happen to get pregnant before being on a good exercise routine, take the time to start slowly and do exercises that aren't going to cause too much strain on the body. Walking and swimming are great for this, as are yoga and other stretching movements.

There are many great reasons to exercise during all phases your life, but it is especially important when you are pregnant. Some of the benefits of working out and getting some regular exercise when you are pregnant or planning on conceiving include:

- Reduces your risk of high blood pressure and gestational diabetes.

- Helps you to get your pre-baby body back faster after birth.

- Makes your labor easier.

- Helps to release happy feelings and alleviates your depression or bad feelings.

- Lifts your spirit.

- Eases any constipation.

- Reduces your stress levels.

- Helps provide better sleep.

- Gives you more energy.

Consider starting an exercise program before getting pregnant so your body is ready to take on the challenges that come with pregnancy and birth. Start out slow and listen to your body to ensure that you are giving it the best care possible. You can slowly add in harder exercises as you get more comfortable with the strain and hard work.

10. Visit your doctor

Before getting pregnant, you should take some time to visit your doctor. They should go through a full check up with you, including a breast check and a pap smear. This is a good way to help you figure out how healthy you are going into the pregnancy and you can discuss with your doctor some of the steps that you can take to prepare your body more for pregnancy before you try to conceive and start the pregnancy.

This is the time when you need to talk to your doctor and ask questions. Your doctor will be able to explain some of the changes that your body will go through and even what you are able to expect while trying to conceive. Your doctor will have your full health history so they can discuss some things that are particular to your body, rather than just general information that pertains to everyone. Make sure to use this time wisely and get a better and clearer understanding of your body.

Preparing your mind and body for pregnancy is the best thing that you can do to ensure that you and your baby are healthy all the way through your nine months.

Chapter 3:
The Amazing Effects of Holistic Medicine on Your Pregnancy

The way that you look at childbirth is going to make a huge difference on how you feel during your pregnancy. While the processes of pregnancy and childbirth are physical, there is so much more to the process than that. In fact, they are major transitions in life. You are going from a life without this child to one with this child. Even if you have had children before, your pregnancy will change your life into a 'before' and an 'after.' The changes that are going to occur during pregnancy and the birth of your child will affect every part of your life, including your beliefs, values, and relationships. This is why it makes so much sense to use a holistic approach during your pregnancy and consider the spirit, mind, and body.

When you are considering getting pregnant, or if you already are pregnant, you are probably trying to figure out the best things to do to have a healthy pregnancy. You want to know how to have the best emotional and physical health as you possibly can during this time. Many mothers even wonder how they can naturally get through labor without too much pain for themselves or stress to the baby. A holistic approach could be the answer that you need to all of these questions, and can give you the best pregnancy possible.

Physical Benefits

First, let's take a look at some of the physical benefits that you can receive when you use a holistic approach for your pregnancy. Pregnancy is a very physical time. You are growing another human being inside of you. This is going to make some huge changes to your body, both those that can be seen, such as your growing belly and swollen ankles, and others that aren't so obvious, such as some common internal discomforts throughout the body.

Using the holistic approach is going to help you to build a good foundation for helping your baby to stay healthy. A physical activity program designed for your personal situation can work in concert with eating a diet that is healthy and full of great nutrients, and can make all the difference in how well your baby grows and how good you feel during the whole pregnancy.

A holistic approach brings a wider range of tools and options to support you through your pregnancy. For example, acupuncture and massage, as long as they are done with someone certified for pregnancy, can help to provide some comfort during this time and will lower your risk of developing some of the more undesirable side effects that show up in some pregnancies. If you are having a lot of trouble during your pregnancy, consider using the holistic approach to find ways to make it a little better.

Emotional Benefits

Having a baby is a very emotional time. While most people expect you to always be happy and excited about your baby, in reality it can be a little bit difficult. Sure, you are excited to bring in a new life into the world and can't wait to meet your newborn, but there are a lot of hormones in play that are going all over the place, making it difficult to just feel happiness and joy all the time.

During pregnancy, you could feel sadness, anxiety, worry, and stress. Add on some of the discomforts that come naturally from the pregnancy, then add on the lack of sleep that comes towards the end of your pregnancy and the beginning of your time as a parent, and you will find that being happy all of the time is pretty much impossible.

When you use the holistic approach, you are going to learn how to acknowledge these emotions, realizing that they are a natural part of your pregnancy. You will be able to work on finding the right strategies to reduce the stress levels and cope in a healthy way with all of the surging emotions as they come up.

When you learn how to cope with stress, you will be able to handle your emotions and feel more in control. You will have more peace of mind, and reduce many of the bad effects that high stress can have on your physical health. When you reduce stress, you will decrease your blood pressure and heart rate, have improved digestion, reduce muscle tension, and enhance your ability to deal with the discomfort and pain of pregnancy.

The first thing that you should work on is finding the best techniques that work for you in order to reduce your levels of stress. There are many options, but you may find one that you like over the others. Some options that work well include yoga, self-hypnosis, meditation, guided imagery, and breath-work. There may be classes or teachers in your area who can help you learn how to make this work during your pregnancy.

After you have learned which technique you like the most, you should work to gain more knowledge. The more you know about your body and how it works both normally, and with differences that occur during a pregnancy, the easier it is to deal with some of the stress that comes up during this time.

Being in charge during this time is important not only for your stress levels, but also for the growth and development of your new baby. You need to gain the right knowledge to ensure that you are picking out the right healthcare provider who will support you, listen to you, and work with you on a holistic approach. You need knowledge to choose which stress relieving techniques are going to work the best for you. Without the proper tools at your disposal, it can become problematic to feel confident as you take care of yourself during pregnancy.

Spiritual Benefits

Not only is pregnancy a time when you are going to see changes in your physical and emotional well-being, but it is also a time when some of your spiritual perspective may change. Many people feel that they grow spiritually when they are pregnant. Growing a new life inside of you can be an intense experience. Then, after marveling at the miracle of birth and becoming a mother, you may find your spiritual connection and awareness becoming stronger in the process.

In addition, any spiritual values and beliefs that you had before are going to come into play even stronger now that you are pregnant and deciding for two. Some people don't like the idea of using medications during labor or going into a hospital for their birth. During pregnancy, you are going to find out how strong your beliefs actually are and they will shape a lot of the decisions that you make during your pregnancy.

During your pregnancy, you should take some time to reflect on the experience. Yes, this may seem a bit difficult with all of the other things that are going on in your life, but take just a few minutes each day to reflect and ponder on your experience and how you feel deep inside during your pregnancy. Ask yourself how you can go even deeper into what you are feeling and find out what is the root of the experience, it may lead you to something greater which will affect you in the long term. Take time to practice meditation, or prayer as part of your reflection time.

Some people find that starting a journal right at the beginning of your pregnancy can be very helpful. As you progress through the pregnancy, you are going to find that it is helpful for relieving stress, and it can help you to understand more fully what it means to be a mother. Plus, it could be a nice keepsake to provide to your baby when they are older and going through a pregnancy of their own.

There are so many aspects of your life that are going to be influenced during your pregnancy. Your body is going to go through a ton of physical changes that others are able to see, and for some, the idea of getting that pre-pregnancy body back will seem impossible. You will feel a wide range of emotions and fears that are hard to deal with, even though everyone expects you to be happy all the time. You may also spend quite a bit of time reflecting on your current and changing beliefs, and learning how they are going to influence your pregnancy.

Learning to embrace all of these aspects of your health is important in ensuring that you have a healthy pregnancy. The holistic approach looks at each one of these to help you make the right decisions for both you and your unborn child. Proponents believe it to be a superior method and one that provides a more natural and organic entry into the world for your baby, as well as a warmer and more supportive pregnancy and childbirth experience for you.

Chapter 4:
Breaking Down Your Pregnancy

Your pregnancy is split up into three trimesters. Each one is important, and means different things for you and for the baby. Each trimester is going to show phases of transition, and you should know that your nutritional needs will change as well. Let's take some time to look through each of the three trimesters and see what changes are in store for your body.

First Trimester

You will be in the first trimester for the first fourteen weeks of your pregnancy. You will likely not know even about the pregnancy for the first two to four weeks, as it starts on the first day of your last menstrual cycle and most women don't realize they are pregnant until they have missed their first menstrual cycle, four weeks later.

This stage of pregnancy is the one where many women will experience morning sickness, although there are women who won't experience this symptom at all. Keep in mind that morning sickness does not just happen in the morning and can in fact happen anytime during the day. Women will also notice that their breasts start to feel sore and enlarged.

The first trimester is a very important time for development of the fetus, and your nutritional intake needs to be optimal. You should use some caution if you consistently use herbal teas, as there are quite a few of them that aren't necessarily safe, and enough research hasn't been done yet to definitively prove how they can affect the fetus. But what is proven however, through many rounds of experience and research, is that eating healthy whole natural non-processed foods and keeping up with a consistent exercise routine will make a huge difference in the development of the baby.

These are some guidelines to follow when you are in your first trimester:

- Keep your diet balanced with lots of fiber, minerals, vitamins, omega fatty acids, antioxidants – we recommend a plant-based diet because plants are the most nutritious and perfect for the human body – save the animals!

- Eat at least 2200 calories a day – if following a plant-based diet, it is recommended to be careful not to under-eat as many plants are low in calories and high in volume. It will be easier to get the calories in by adding fatty foods to your diet like nuts, seeds and avocado. Eat lots, you are eating for two!

- Pick out a good prenatal vitamin.

- Do not use tobacco or alcohol during any part of your pregnancy.

- Keep up with your exercise program unless directed not to by your doctor.

- Keep hydrated at all times of the day, and avoid getting overheated.

A regular routine of stretching and light aerobic exercise will make your pregnancy and childbirth experience easier and more enjoyable.

Another benefit of exercise is how it can strengthen your muscles. This helps to reduce some of the stretching that happens while you are carrying the baby. In addition, the muscles will be stronger, making it easier to get through labor without as much pain, and shortening the amount of time it takes for the baby to be born.

Second Trimester

This stage of the pregnancy goes from the 14th week until the end of your seventh month. Many women find that this is the easiest part of the pregnancy. Some of your energy that was lost during the first trimester is going to return and you won't suffer as much from the morning sickness, although there are a few women who will still feel these symptoms. Towards the end of the second trimester, you will notice that your belly is expanding and you will eventually start to feel the baby moving around and kicking.

During this time, you will be responsible for eating a healthy diet, and you should start increasing your caloric intake a bit. Most women will be advised to take in an additional 300 calories a day, unless they are carrying multiples. Increasing your caloric intake is going to make a huge difference in the health of your baby.

Things to consider during your second trimester:

- Increase intake to at least 2500 calories each day.

- Continue to maintain a diet that is well-balanced and high in nutrients. Completely eliminate unhealthy food choices.

- Continue taking your prenatal vitamins.

- Continue avoiding all alcohol and tobacco.

- Modify your exercise program in order to protect the stomach, back, and weight bearing muscles.

- Be careful when carrying or lifting heavy items because your weight is now distributed differently, causing your balance to shift.

During this trimester, it is common for an expecting mother to have some issues with their digestive systems. Keep track of those foods that seem to bother you and avoid them as much as possible.

This is the time of the pregnancy when the baby really starts to grow. Most mothers will get to see the gender of their baby if they choose, and even feel the baby move during this stage. But as the baby keeps growing, the stomach is going have less room, which can cause indigestion and gas. To help prevent this issue, you should consider eating your food slowly and go with smaller meals and snacks. Also, drink more liquids to help with this issue and to prevent any hydration issues.

Third Trimester

This stage is going to last until the time the baby is delivered. The baby is going to triple in weight, making things more difficult on the mother. You will need to get in enough calories to take care of you and the baby, but you will need to be careful about when and how you do it. Consider snacking and smaller meals to ensure that you aren't overfilling the stomach or causing other discomfort in your pregnancy.

During this stage, you are going to see even more changes in your body. You may be more anxious and emotional. You may notice an awkwardness and new discomfort as you adjust to a body that is changing so dramatically. Get plenty of rest and relaxation as needed.

There are many great tips that you can follow to make your final trimester a bit easier.

- Continue eating at least 2500 calories.

- Eat more frequent and smaller meals to avoid discomfort and heartburn.

- Continue taking your prenatal vitamins.

- Continue avoiding alcohol and tobacco.

- Keep track of the hydration that you are taking in. Keep a water bottle near you all the time, so you and the baby are healthy and getting plenty of water each day.

- Change up the exercise regimen that you are using to ensure that your joints and muscles are staying healthy and that you are not overdoing it, or risking injury.

- Reduce some of the intensity of your workouts since shortness of breath can become common in this stage. Do not become too winded at this time.

- Practice toning and stretching to get ready for childbirth.

This final stage of pregnancy is an important one. It is the last few months that you have before you bring that little bundle of joy into the world. Take some time to relax and get things organized so you can put all of your attention into your little one when they finally arrive.

Chapter 5:
Keeping That Baby Growing—Healthy Habits Every Mother Should Know

During your pregnancy, you need to carefully figure out the best habits for keeping you and the baby as healthy as possible. Here are some of the healthy habits that you should try out to have the best pregnancy possible through all stages.

Healthy Breakfast

Even if you were not a big breakfast eater before your pregnancy, you should start eating breakfast now. Consider eating something, even if it is small, so that you can get some nutrients into the baby. You should avoid all junk food and processed un-natural products; rather, choose things with lots of nutrients, such as fruits or veggies, and see the difference in how good you feel – your baby will thank you one day.

Plenty of Sleep

Sleep during pregnancy is really important. Of course, it is one of the hardest things to do when you are pregnant because of the new shape of your body, the discomfort associated with your big belly, and how much the baby is going to move around. Don't give up on getting good quality restorative sleep. It is very important for both you and your baby.

So how much sleep do you need to get to stay healthy? Most research finds that if you don't get at least 6 hours of sleep each night, you are not going to be getting enough. As an expecting mother, you will often need more than this minimum since your body is going through more stress than normal. We recommend sleeping at least 8 or 9 hours at night, and even an hour or two during the day.

Some of the steps that you can take to get plenty of sleep into your daily schedule include:

- Get to bed early. Try to adjust to the cycle of the sun and moon for a healthy circadian rhythm.

- When you have to get up at night to use the bathroom, get it done quickly and get straight back to bed. Avoid things that will wake you up more and make it more difficult to get back to sleep.

- Avoid snacking before bed, especially sweet fruit and grains because the raised blood sugar can inhibit your sleep.

- Keep the room dark. Any light can interrupt your circadian rhythm and result in poor rest during the night.

- Keep the room cool. While most people keep their rooms warm, this can make it harder to sleep. Don't let the temperature get above 70 degrees during the night.

- Do not watch TV or browse online before bed as this can keep the mind engaged, making it difficult to fall asleep.

Use a Probiotic

Probiotics are one of the best things that you can consume during your pregnancy. These are known as the friendly bacteria required to keep the body healthy and functional. Some of the benefits of probiotics include:

- Preventing premature labor.

- Preventing skin and food allergies in your baby.

- Preventing inflammatory bowel disease.

- Preventing bacterial vaginosis.

- Preventing recurrent bladder and ear infections.

Add Exercise

No one would advise a pregnant woman to train for a marathon, but that doesn't mean that women should refrain from all exercise during pregnancy. Many worry that extra movement is bad for the mother and baby, and that mothers should be resting so as not to cause harm.

Anything, when taken to the extreme, can cause problems. As long as you listen to your body and continue on with your regular exercise program, it can be really beneficial to you and the baby during the pregnancy. It can help to keep your body strong while carrying the baby. It can make labor easier and shorter. It can even help to alleviate your bad moods and make you feel happier when you otherwise might tend to feel sad or when your hormones are all over the map.

Consider doing 30 minutes or so of moderate activity each day. If you were doing an exercise program before you got pregnant, you should be able to continue with this same one, as long as you get permission from your doctor and listen to your body. If the activity is too tough, slow it down or try something else to keep safe during this time.

There are a few exercises that you should be careful about. Keep away from floor exercises. These are hard on the back because of all of the excess weight from the baby. Balancing workouts are not the best because these can cause harm if the mother falls. Any workout such as martial arts or kickboxing should be avoided because the stomach could get harmed while participating.

There are many other exercises that you could consider that are safe and healthy for both the mother and the baby. These include:

- Walking.

- Swimming.

- Yoga.

- Dancing.

- Stretching.

- Light jogging.

- Easy weight lifting.

For the most part, if you were doing an activity before you became pregnant, you will be able to continue on with it during the pregnancy. Just make some adjustments to the workout to go with your stage of the pregnancy so you aren't overstretching the muscles and causing unneeded harm to you and the baby. Always listen to your body to find out the right intensity and activity level that will help you keep your heart strong without pain or discomfort.

Make sure to talk to your doctor about your exercise routine before getting started. They can give you some guidance on what to do for your workouts and will discuss with you any potential issues that you may face and should be aware of. If at any time something hurts or doesn't feel right, make sure to stop and relax.

Chapter 6:
Eating for Two:—How to Eat Healthy While Pregnant

The food choices you make will never as important as when you are pregnant. Not only are you trying to get enough nutrition to keep yourself healthy, but you need nutrition to keep the baby growing and developing as well.

Nutrition Throughout the Pregnancy

There are some important nutrients that you must get into the body when you are trying to stay healthy, no matter which stage of pregnancy you are in. You should include enough calories, fats, and protein. First, let's look at the calories. You are eating the food that is needed for both you and a new baby, but this does not mean you need to eat double your daily calorie allowance. During the first trimester, you should consume an extra 100 to 300 calories every day. Later in the pregnancy, you can bump this up to 450 to 500 calories extra.

If you are pregnant with multiples, your healthcare provider may have some other rules that you should follow regarding your calorie count. Make sure to listen and find out the best amount for your needs.

The most important nutrients for pregnancy include:

- Protein—the amount that you will need should increase as the baby starts to grow. You will need to expand your consumption by at least 25 grams by the third trimester.

- Vitamin D—this nutrient helps prevent hyperparathyroidism, helps the bones to stay strong, and helps the digestive system. You can get this from a supplement and the sun. There are many reasons you could be low on vitamin D, so make sure to get in as much sunlight as you can.

- Iron—you will need a lot more iron during your pregnancy. Without the right amount, you and the baby will suffer with issues including hypothyroidism, low weight gain for the mother and low birth weight in the baby. Take in at least 27 mg. of iron every day.

- Folate—this nutrient is good for fetal growth. It is an enzyme that is good for the right development of your neural tubes. You should start taking some folate before you get pregnant, at least 400 to 1000 mcg each day, to ensure that you are getting enough. Continue taking folate if breastfeeding as well. Liver, citrus fruits, green vegetables, and spinach all contain folate.

- Essential fatty acids—these are the starters for other fatty acids that need to be made to keep the body healthy. Consider eating some hemp seeds or flax seeds – they are rich with essential fatty acids.

- Vitamin C and bioflavonoids—these work to protect the capillaries and the veins while carrying the baby. Eat plenty of fresh fruits to get a lot of vitamin C and bioflavonoids in your system.

- Calcium—make sure that you are getting at least 1200 mg of calcium each day. If you do not take in enough calcium, you could have issues with eclampsia and hypertension. Calcium can also protect you from lead toxicity.

- Magnesium—this works with the calcium in your body to help ensure that it is absorbed properly, your pH levels are regulated, and you have the right balance of electrolytes.

Recommended Daily Nutrients

Some recommendations for proper nutrient intake during your healthy pregnancy include:

Protein—60 to 100 grams.

Calories—2300.

Vitamin A—2565 to 5000 IU.

Vitamin D—5 to 10 mcg.

Vitamin C—80 to 85 mg.

Manganese—2 mg.

Copper—1 mg.

Chromium—30 mcg.

Iodine—175 to 220 mcg.

Zinc—11 to 20 mg.

Iron—27 to 60 mg.

Magnesium 350 to 450 mg.

Phosphorus—700 to 1200 mg.

Calcium—1000-1200 mg.

Vitamin B12—2.6 to 4 mcg.

Folic Acid—400 to 800 mcg.

Vitamin B6—1.9 to 2.6 mg.

Niacin—15 to 18 mg.

Vitamin B2—1.4 to 1.5 mg.

Vitamin B1—1.4 mg.

Vitamin E—15 mg.

Keep in mind that you do not have to get these amounts exact each day. Stressing out about missing something small is not going to make you feel better, it will most likely make you feel worse. Stress does more damage to your body than nutrient deficiency!

Chapter 7:
Herbal Supplementation to Boost Your Pregnancy

You should always use caution when it comes to picking out the herbs that you are going to use. While many of these may seem safe because they are all natural, the side effects can cause damage to both mother and baby. Make sure to discuss the herb you plan to use with your doctor to ensure that you are doing what is best for you and for your baby during the pregnancy.

If you and your doctor determine that using a certain herb is fine, make sure that you are doing so in a way that is safe. Recommendations include:

- When you first start, use herbs that are gentle. Never use a plant that is considered toxic during your pregnancy.

- Only work with one herb at a time. Then if something feels off, you know which one is to blame.

- Invest in a book or guide which can help you to select and identify the plants you may use.

Morning Sickness

If your morning sickness is really bad and nothing seems to be working, try out this herbal remedy; drink a cup of fennel or anise seed tea right when you wake up. If you are feeling the morning sickness later in the day, sip a cup of spearmint or peppermint infusion.

Backache

A common complaint that many pregnant women will deal with is aches in their back. You are carrying around more weight than you are used to and this could cause stress to your back as well as some of the other organs in the body as the pregnancy progresses.

Magnesium and calcium are good at helping to minimize and prevent backaches, and you can find these in foods such as nuts, seeds, figs, apples, and green vegetables. Consider some wheat grass as well since it has many nutrients that are great for calming the nerves, nourishing the muscles, and helping the spine to stay strong. Heat, such as a warm shower or bath, and a nice rub can help to relieve the tension and keep your back strong.

Heartburn

Heartburn is a common complaint for many pregnant women.

Some of the things you can try include:

- Fennel or anise seed tea.

- Papaya and pineapple after your meals can help because of the enzymes that help to digest the food.

- Frequent small meals instead of fewer large ones.

- Don't lay down right after eating.

Recommended Herbs

Herbs recommended for use during pregnancy:

- Alfalfa—this one has digestive enzymes, iron, calcium, carotenoids, and many great vitamins. These are good for avoiding hemorrhage and anemia when you are giving birth.

- Burdock root—this one is full of minerals that are good for keeping the liver strong, supporting the urinary organs, stimulating digestion, works as a laxative, and balances your blood sugar.

- Dandelion root and leaves—strengthens the bladder and kidneys, and works wonders on your digestive tract.

- Ginger root—this one is good to use when you are suffering from morning sickness. Good for the chills and helping out with your circulation.

- Kelp—lots of minerals and vitamins that are good for the pregnant body.

- Lavender—good to put in teas to help calm down nerves, lift a depressed mood, and promote sleep. It is good for relieving gas and indigestion as well.

- Lemon balm—promotes digestion, reduces tension, and can calm down the nerves.

- Motherwort—this is a good one to strengthen your heart while reducing your stress and treating some hypertension as long as it is taken after the first trimester.

- Partridge berry—this is a good one for the nervous system and your uterine systems.

- St. John's Wort—this is good as an external oil and it works for sciatica, sore back, and any aching muscles that occur while the baby is growing. You can also use it internally for nerve pain, depression, and infections.

- Rose hips—this one is high in vitamin C so it is good for the circulatory and immune system.

- Red raspberry leaves—lots of minerals and vitamins. Helps to tone up the muscles of the uterus and will work to prevent hemorrhaging during childbirth.

- Yellow dock—good for many issues such as skin health, hormone balance, digestion, and constipation. It is also good for supporting the health of your liver.

These are just a few of the herbs that you can consider if you would like to get the most out of your pregnancy without worrying about taking harmful medications. Make sure to discuss the use of these herbs with your doctor before getting started to ensure you will not hinder other pregnancy issues that you and your baby are dealing with. But for most pregnancies, these are going to be safe and effective for you to use.

If you have never used some of these herbs in the past, you should be careful. Remember that you should only take in one herb at a time. This allows you to figure out if there are issues with allergies and cease using the herb if it isn't good for you. Never take anything that has known side effects towards the pregnancy or you risk harming yourself and the baby. Talk to your doctor if you are uncertain about any herbal remedies.

Chapter 8:
Keeping Baby Safe—Things to
Avoid During Pregnancy

Pregnancy is a normal part of life, and one can experience it without drastically changing their life routine, however, there are some known hazards that should be avoided.

Processed Foods and Sugar

During pregnancy, you should develop the discipline to stay away from processed foods and sugars. Sure, these seem to be just what your cravings are wanting at the time and they sound so good, and are easy to make, but they are bad for your body.

Make sure to stay away from artificial sweeteners.

Many people who are on diets or who are trying to be healthier will choose to go with artificial sweeteners, thinking these are better than other options. In reality, they are even worse for your health! Artificial sweeteners can be very harmful to the body, and have been found to cause brain tumors, migraines, and depression.

There are some safe sweeteners that you can choose from instead that will help you sweeten up your food without all the negative impact. Stevia and Xylitol are the best options and can even provide you with some health benefits! For example, xylitol is good for stronger bones, fewer cavities, fewer infections, and better gum health.

Caffeine

This one is really hard for a lot of new mothers. They are used to having some coffee in the morning or soda in the afternoon to help keep them awake through the day. Now that they are really needing the energy boost, they are told that caffeine is not allowed.

While some doctors will allow a little bit of caffeine on occasion, you will need to be careful about the consumption. Caffeine is addictive and it can pass over to the developing baby. This may be a good time to point out that after the baby is born, mothers still must pay careful attention to what they put in their bodies, because whatever they ingest, goes straight through the breast milk and into the baby.

If you would like to get some of the same feelings that you did with a soda before your pregnancy, while still getting rid of your caffeine content, consider using sparkling water. This gives you the bubbles and could trick your mind into thinking it gets a treat. Adding flavor like some fresh lemon is fine as long as you aren't adding in any sugar.

Alcohol

It is never recommended to consume any alcohol during your pregnancy and if you have a dependency on alcohol, it is important to get the right support as soon as possible. While some doctors tell patients not to worry about drinking in the first month of pregnancy because they didn't know about the baby, if you are planning on getting pregnant, stop drinking to be on the safe side for the sake of the baby.

Heavy drinking at any point of the pregnancy can have some far reaching effects on the baby. Some of the birth defects that are believed to be caused by heavy drinking during pregnancy include:

- Physical defects of the organs, face, and heart.

- Behavioral problems.

- Emotional problems.

- Learning problems.

- Mental retardation.

- Increased risk of miscarriage.

- Higher risk of a low birthweight.

- Stillbirth.

Fetal alcohol spectrum disorder is the term that is used most often to describe the umbrella of problems that can happen to the baby when alcohol is consumed during pregnancy.

Smoking

Smoking has been proven to have negative impacts on unborn babies and should be avoided during pregnancy. If you are planning on getting pregnant, make sure that you stop smoking before you try to conceive. If you get pregnant unexpectedly, stop smoking immediately.

Babies who are born to mothers who smoked are likely to weigh less. This could be due to the fact that there is less blood flow, so fewer nutrients are able to make it to the baby.

Anti-bacterial Soaps

These kinds of soaps can have some issues impacting the health of your baby. While these were popular for some time, there are now tests which show they don't offer much in terms of protection against the germs they claim to help with. In fact, some new studies have shown that these soaps are actually able to form carcinogens when they are mixed together with water. This is terrible for your pregnancy, and even after birth.

Cell Phones

While it is not practical to drop the use of your phone when you are pregnant, you should be careful with how much you use it. A new study has found that women who used their phone in excess each day were more likely to have children who grew up with behavioral issues.

The less you are around the harmful radiation of cell phones during the pregnancy, the better health the baby will have as well. Try using headphones when speaking on the phone and keep the phone off and away when you are going to sleep. Limit your cell phone use as much as possible.

Other Things to Avoid

Some of the other things that you may need to consider avoiding during pregnancy, or should at least discuss with your doctor, include:

- Microwaving your food—it is a bad idea to microwave food, period. It can interfere with the chemical structure of your food and can make the food harder to digest. It is best to heat food on a pan or pot.

- Avoid dairy—some women are fine with eating dairy, but some may be sensitive to it. Eating dairy when you are sensitive is hard on the baby and could increase the risk of dairy allergies, throat and ear infections, and asthma.

- Too much vitamin A—while this vitamin is important in pregnancy, taking too much could cause birth defects and other issues with your baby's development.

- Soy—some people believe that soy can be hazardous during pregnancy and even with breastfeeding. Discuss this with your doctor.

Cleanse With Water

During pregnancy, you need to cleanse your body. This means drinking plenty of pure water. You should not go with distilled or tap water because there can be many harmful chemicals and heavy metals inside. Instead, choose to go with filtered or spring water.

Tap water can have fluoride, arsenic, and chlorine inside, as well as chemicals that can be toxic and could damage your body. According to the U.S. Environmental Protection Agency, there have been samples of water through the country that contain even anti-depressants, birth control, and antibiotics.

The most important thing you can do regarding the water your baby drinks, is to understand where it really comes from. Water testing results are a matter of public record, so you may not need to rely only on what you are told. Educate yourself and act accordingly.

Household Chemicals

There are many household cleaners that you may be using in your home that have harmful toxins. Some of the chemicals that you should be careful around and avoid include:

- Toilet bowl cleaners.

- Window cleaners.

- Pesticides and insecticides.

- Varnish and paint.

- Paint stripper.

- Air fresheners.

- White spirit or turpentine.

- Aerosols.

- Dry cleaning fluid.

- Carpet cleaner.

- Bleach.

While these are harmful, you do need to keep your home clean. Consider using products that are made with 100% natural non-toxic ingredients or go with vinegar. Vinegar is effective and isn't going to harm you during pregnancy. You can use it to sanitize or disinfect any surface, so it is perfect for your whole home.

Some other options that you can use to keep the home clean and healthy include lemon juice, salt and baking soda.

Plastic Exposure

Being exposed to phthalates, an ingredient that is found inside of plastic, could be an issue for birth defects and could even make your pregnancy end sooner. Some chemicals that are released into the environment, all coming from plastic, are causing male humans and male animals to be born with feminine characteristics instead.

It is common for a woman to come into contact with these chemicals. They are found inside common items such as:

- Insect repellants.

- Hairsprays.

- Nail polishes.

- Moisturizers.

- Food containers.

Ingesting, inhaling, and absorbing these chemicals can cause a variety of problems, including fertility issues. It is best to avoid these chemicals as much as possible in all stages of your life.

It is highly believed that plastic exposure, especially with these toxins, is the biggest reason that male infertility has gone so high. Plus, research has shown that now we are statistically seeing fewer males being born today compared to years ago. Many believe that these high levels of exposure to plastics could be the root cause.

Teflon and BPA can cause many of the same issues, so learn how to avoid these as much as possible for the best results for you and for the healthy life of your unborn baby.

Lead

Your doctor will test your baby by the time they reach the age of one for lead poisoning. While most toy manufacturers have removed lead from their products, you should be careful with old toys as some of them may still contain lead and not be in the wave of new manufacturing.

Many old homes will have lead inside. Paint used to be made out of lead and this could cause harm if you or the baby ingest any of the paint. Have your home tested for lead and consider switching out the paint to avoid any issues or risk.

Lead can cause a lot of harmful effects to the body, especially for your baby. It can be toxic, causing birth defects, developmental issues and much more.

Chapter 9:
Avoiding Danger and Pain—Natural and Pain Free Ways to Get Through Childbirth

Your pregnancy is a major milestone in your life. Your mind is affected, your body is going to change like crazy, and you are going to notice that your emotions are changing. Everything about your body and about your life will be different from the moment that you find out that you are pregnant.

Because pregnancy has so much to do with your overall health and how your life goes, the holistic approach is perfect for helping you and the baby be healthy throughout this process. When you use a holistic approach in your pregnancy, you are choosing a lifestyle that is going to help labor progress as naturally as possible.

Prepares You with Information

It is really hard to choose the right path and treatment for yourself if you don't have all the facts. You will work with your doctor to learn what things enhance the process of labor. If you are well informed ahead of time, you will be able to understand and make good decisions regarding your consent to what your doctor or midwife is proposing. This is empowering and gives the mother a lot of confidence knowing she can make these decisions.

When you choose the holistic approach, you will learn about the various risks and benefits of all childbirth options. While most holistic doctors may choose to go with the natural progression of labor, they will also talk about some of the other childbirth options in case labor does not go as planned.

For example, your doctor may feel that your labor needs to be induced for the health of the baby or because you have gone too far past your due date. You will then learn about some of the options that come with induction so you can discuss the plan and decide whether or not this is the right decision for you. You will learn about which induction methods will provide the most support while minimizing the need for intervention.

In some cases your doctor may recommend a caesarean section, even though you had wished for a natural labor. If the baby is breech or there are other medical concerns, natural labor may not be best for your baby. With the holistic approach, it is often recommended to let the mother go through natural labor first, since babies who do so have been shown to have better lung functioning. But in some cases your doctor may decide the risk is too high and will begin the surgery before any natural labor can occur.

Avoid Unneeded Technology Use

There is a lot of technology used in labor today that is not necessary. Vacuum extractors, forceps, and some fetal monitoring are all choices of the past and could actually harm the baby. Very rarely will you need these, but some doctors will choose to use them simply to speed up the process, rather than because they are necessary, at the expense of your labor and the health of the baby.

When you are talking to your doctor or midwife, ask about their use of these items. Most holistic practitioners are not going to use them unless absolutely necessary because of the complications that they can introduce.

The holistic approach tends to focus more time and attention on the patient and there tends to be much less commercialization in these medical practices.

Pain Management

Pain management is something that all expecting mothers worry about. Labor is difficult in the best of cases, and women who have opted for a holistic delivery are sometimes fearful that they will get into hard labor, then not have access to options to ease their pain. There are a number of options that you can choose from with the holistic approach, including self-hypnosis, hydrotherapy, movement, breathing, and guided imagery.

Don't worry, you do not have to give birth without medication if you so choose. These holistic options can be used in addition to traditional labor options like the epidural.

The reason that many people are choosing the holistic alternatives is because of the high risks that come from pain medications. Some risks that you may have when using an epidural during childbirth that are not present with alternative treatments include:

- You are using medications that are narcotics. These can prolong your labor, interfere with how well you can move around, cause nausea, and make you lightheaded and groggy. None of this is good through the labor process.

- Babies born using these medications can be sleepy and may need breathing stimulation. This could also interfere with breastfeeding in the hospital.

- Some studies show that epidurals increase the need for caesarean sections.

- These medications can lower blood pressure, and in effect, drop how much oxygen is getting to your baby during the labor process.

- Backaches, infections, itching, and even permanent damage to the nerves can all occur, especially if the epidural is put in improperly at the time of childbirth.

While it is still possible to use medications during labor when using the holistic approach, the idea is to limit their use. Other options can be tried first and in many cases will be successful.

The amount of medication used can be reduced with the use of tools like breathing and guided imagery, in addition to some of the other holistic techniques. With less time on the medication and less medication being used, it will be so much safer for you and for the baby.

This method of childbirth can help to reduce the amount of technology that you will use while also reducing how much medication is necessary for the labor. Talk through this process with your doctor before making any decisions so you are informed and can make a good concrete plan for the end of your pregnancy.

Chapter 10:
Kicking Pregnancy Discomfort
to the Curb

During your pregnancy, you are going to notice that there is a lot of discomfort that goes on as the baby grows and begins to develop more and more. Some mothers go through so much pain and discomfort that they elect to have the baby come early. It is not recommended to do this though; your baby needs to grow until at least 39 weeks to ensure they are fully ready to grow on their own. Luckily, you do not need to suffer through the discomforts; there are many holistic therapies that you can use to alleviate the aches and pains and make it to the end of your pregnancy.

Morning Sickness

This discomfort is one that many women experience and it can be challenging since you know that you must give your baby the proper nutrition, even though you can barely keep your food down. Most women find that an empty stomach can make morning sickness even worse so you should learn to space snacks to avoid this issue. Some other things that you can try out for your morning sickness problems include:

- Eat some crackers—go for some with a bit of salt before getting out of bed to help fill your stomach.

- Drink between meals—water during meals can actually be hard on the pregnant belly. Drink before and after meals, rather than during the meals.

- Snack at night—while you may have been told this is bad for your health, having a little fruit at night, perhaps on your way back from the bathroom, can ensure that your blood sugars are stabilized and you won't get sick in the morning. Don't have too much however, otherwise it may be difficult to go back to sleep.

- Try some sea sickness options. Don't go for the pills, but try pressure bracelets, they can do wonders for alleviating some of the worse symptoms that come with morning sickness.

For most moms, the morning sickness is going to start going away by the beginning of the second trimester. If your morning sickness is really severe and you can't keep any food down, or it lasts well into the second trimester, make sure to discuss this with your doctor.

Backaches

Another common issue that a lot of mothers will deal with is backaches. The baby weighs a lot and can put extra stress on your back as they continue to grow. A few things that you can do to help alleviate some of this pain in pregnancy include:

- Good posture—make sure to stand and sit up nice and tall at all times.

- Lifting—as your stomach gets bigger, your lifting should decrease. If you do need to pick something up, bend with your knees rather than at the waist.

- Good shoes—shoes that have a lot of support and a low heel are best.

- Sit down—standing, especially standing still, puts a lot of pressure on your back. If you need to stand for long periods, bring out a stool to rest one of your feet, switching back and forth, to relieve some of this stress while standing.

- Exercise—this can help strengthen all those back muscles.

- Massages, warm baths, hot water bottles, and plenty of rest can help as well.

If none of these are working for you, talk to your doctor about other remedies you can try. Do not take painkillers and other medications as these can be hard on the baby.

Headache

With all the hormonal changes and higher blood volume, some women do get headaches. These can also be increased due to tension, anxiety, eyestrain, fatigue, and stuffy noses. Some suggestions that can limit headaches include:

- Learn what triggers the headaches so you can avoid these triggers when possible.

- Cool washcloths or ice packs on the head or neck.

- Get more sleep and consider adding in a nap when possible.

- Get in enough liquids as dehydration can be a cause.

- Find time to relax with massages or a nice bath.

- Get fresh air each day.

Headaches can appear for a variety of different reasons. Make sure you figure out what is causing yours and learn how you can make it go away. If the issue is not going away on its own, make sure to bring this up with your doctor.

Mood Changes

Pregnancy is a time of many mood changes. You could be happy one second and then mad and upset the next. The changes in your hormones, stress, and fatigue can all be to blame. Some things you can do to handle these mood changes include:

- Talk about your feelings with someone you can trust.

- Join a pregnancy support group so you can share your experience with others.

- Do things that you enjoy. Just because you are pregnant doesn't mean you shouldn't take care of yourself in the process.

- Pamper yourself. Before the baby comes, take time to get your hair done or do your nails or something else that is just for yourself to brighten your mood.

- Get enough exercise. This is a great way to lift those blues and has been shown to help alleviate depression and keep the mood in a consistent place.

- Don't get too tired. Try to take some naps, even 15 minutes, when possible.

- Eat a healthy diet. An unhealthy diet, can set you up to be in a really grumpy mood.

- Include plenty of iron and protein into your diet each day for best results.

- Learn as much as possible about your pregnancy. Read some books, talk to others, and go to classes. Often, knowing as much as possible about pregnancy can help to alleviate some of the tension you may be feeling.

Keep in mind that your emotions are going through a lot at this point in your life and even though you try a few of these options, they are not always going to work. Take the time to do something for yourself, have some fun, and learn how to alleviate some of that pressure and the moodiness may not get quite so bad.

As you can see, there are many natural ways that you can cure some of the most common ailments that come up during a pregnancy.

Conclusion

Thank you again for downloading this book!

I hope we were able to help you to understand the holistic approach and why it is so **important** to the overall health of you and your baby. Most people just don't understand what the whole holistic philosophy is all about, and it's a real shame because if they did, their world would shift in such positive ways!

Many mothers feel that it is too extreme not to follow the mainstream advice of hospitals and painkillers, and it is going to only work if the mother and baby are healthy already. Some women are fearful of the **natural way of living** because it is new to them, therefore they block themselves from the possibility of being healthy. Society tends to mold the masses however is best for the economy, and unfortunately the major corporations don't always have our personal health and best interest in mind.

The holistic approach is more than just about how to carry out a successful and healthy pregnancy. **It is about a lifestyle**, and a way of thinking. It is about becoming more mindful and aware in everything that you do, and by making actions that support mother earth instead of destroy her, we are collectively changing the world to become a better place.

Don't stop here. Keep learning, **keep exploring**, and stay open to the wonderful possibilities and doors opening every day of your life.

We wish you a beautiful pregnancy and delivery!

Free Bonus eBook Access:
15 Homemade Natural After-Birth Remedies

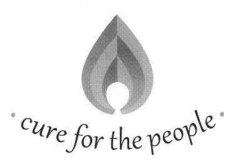

We really hope you enjoyed reading this book, and we want you to know that **we care about our community and the people in it**. That's why we began our collective called 'Cure For The People'. We love to publish lots of different content on various subjects from health to self-help, and much more. We want to open the minds and hearts of our readers, to spread awareness on important topics and have a good time doing it! However, we cannot do what we love to do... without you! Community is the most important part of this movement, and **we want you** to be a part of it!

We would love for you to interact with us and other like-minded individuals on our social media pages, as well as read more great articles and blogs on various related topics, and even get **free chapters from our other books** – all to be found on our website:

www.cure4people.com

You can also find more of our books and video trailers on Amazon which we know **you will LOVE,** by simply visiting our Amazon Author page:

www.amazon.com/author/cure4people

And one last, final thing...

Like we said earlier, community is the most important element required to continue spreading awesome life-changing information to the world – and so if we want people to discover and learn, we need people to trust us and our books! If you could be so kind and helpful, could you please leave us an **honest review** on our Amazon page for this book? We made it super easy and provided the link right here:

www.amazon.com/review/create-review

We give you our big thanks in advance for this super-awesome favor!

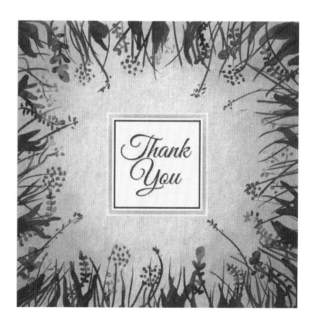

As a big 'THANK YOU' we have written a free bonus eBook, *just for you*. It's an eBook that has no availability or access anywhere but right here. As an even bigger bonus, when you download the free book, you will be subscribed to our newsletter which will continue to provide you **additional valuable content** on this particular subject. We want to continue supporting our readers by engaging with them after they read our books and this is the perfect way to stay connected.

So.. for the moment we have all been waiting for... We present to you... your free bonus ebook:

"15 Homemade Natural After-Birth Remedies"

www.cure4people.com/pregnancy-bonus-938

We hope you enjoy this free content, and we wish to continue our relationship through our newsletter, social media channels, website and blog.

Best Wishes from the Cure For The People family!

Made in the USA
Middletown, DE
14 June 2019